GW01453131

Yoga With a Purpose

How to Unlock Your True Potential & Build a Life of Meaning Through Yoga

Olivia Summers

Published in The USA by:

Success Life Publishing

Hillsborough, NC 27278

Copyright © 2015 by Olivia Summers

ISBN-10: 1512231665

ALL RIGHTS RESERVED. No part of this publication may be reproduced or transmitted in any form whatsoever, electronic, or mechanical, including photocopying, recording, or by any informational storage or retrieval system without the express written permission of the author, except for the use of brief quotations in a book review.

Disclaimer

Every effort has been made to accurately represent this book and its potential. Results vary with every individual, and your results may or may not be different from those depicted. No promises, guarantees or warranties, whether stated or implied, have been made that you will produce any specific result from this book. Your efforts are individual and unique, and may vary from those shown. Your success depends on your efforts, background and motivation.

The material in this publication is provided for educational and informational purposes only and is not intended as medical advice. The information contained in this book should not be used to diagnose or treat any illness, metabolic disorder, disease or health problem. Always consult your physician or health care provider before beginning any nutrition or exercise program. Use of the programs, advice, and information contained in this book is at the sole choice and risk of the reader.

Table of Contents

Introduction

I'm so happy that you decided to pick up this book and start reading it. By doing so, you must inherently know that there's something just slightly *off* about modern yoga practice—that something is missing.

If you're just starting out on your yoga journey and you're reading this, then I'm impressed. It took me much longer to realize that something was missing in my yoga practice and that it wasn't just about postures and the food groups you do or don't eat.

I admit, in my early days of yoga (over 10 years ago!) I was mostly in it for vanity's sake. I mean, who doesn't want to be effortlessly sexy, look younger and feel the best they ever have? I know I wanted that. Especially after gaining the Freshman 15 I was warned about by my mother. So, when the opportunity came for me to take my first yoga class my freshman year of college, I jumped at the chance. But I must admit: it wasn't the magical pill I thought it was going to be.

Don't get me wrong: I *loved* yoga from the start—it was just for all the wrong reasons. I wasn't so much interested in the spiritual side of the practice or becoming a better person. I wanted to be flexible and look hot in a bikini again. Now, I'm not saying that you can't have ulterior motives when you first start out on your yoga journey. Most of us do and that's okay. As long as you start I don't think there's any *wrong* way to find your true path.

But the funny thing about yoga is, it becomes what you need it to be most. Obviously that's going to look different for different people—that's the beauty of it and what I love most about yoga. And if you stick with your journey long enough, eventually you'll start to realize that it's more than you ever thought it could be. I mean that in the most *un*-cliché way possible. But it's true! My love for yoga has grown and evolved in ways that I never dreamed of—it has molded me into a better person than I would be otherwise a million times over.

I'll say it again, though: yoga is **no** magic pill. To find your true calling and wisdom along your path to enlightenment it takes a commitment to look deep within yourself and the ability to be honest about who you are and who you want to *really* be.

So was my 19-year-old self completely and utterly ridiculous for choosing to practice yoga for vanity's sake? Yes. And no. I'm so inherently thankful to the Universe for pulling me in the direction it did when I was just a naïve freshman (is that redundant?). See, I believe in cosmic destiny. That things that are meant to happen do—even if that means we have to be tricked into doing them. Eventually everything gets sorted out and we end up where we're supposed to be.

So even if you just started yoga a week ago, haven't started at all, or have been practicing for a decade, don't be too hard on yourself. I think we're all right where we were meant to be. Remember: it's not a race and there really is no end point. As long as you keep the fire within you alive and are committed to becoming a better version of yourself then you'll undoubtedly discover your true potential and purpose in this life and beyond.

Keep reading to find out how yoga can help you unlock the door to the path of enlightenment.

Who Was Patanjali And
Why Should I Care?

Whether you've been practicing yoga for a month or 5 years—there are some things we need to go over. You may or may not be familiar with the history of yoga, but I'm sure you've heard of Patanjali. He wrote the *Yoga Sutras*. You know, basically the Bible of yoga.

Patanjali himself wasn't the inventor of yoga per se. He just put it all into words—very detailed ones, I might add. His *Sutras* (which means, 'thread') brought together all of the major practices and philosophies of yoga that we know and love today and is thought to have been composed around 400 CE.

Ancient yogic texts might not seem that relevant or important to you, but they hold the secrets to the foundation for a life of meaning and purpose.

Patanjali (and most Hindus for that matter) believed that yoga was much more than just a bunch of postures. In fact, Patanjali laid out a whole system to follow for enlightenment—known as the Eight Limbs of Yoga, or ashtanga (which translates to 'eight limb').

The Eight-Limbed Path

Yamas: how you treat the world

Niyamas: how you treat yourself

Asanas: yoga postures

Pranayama: breathing techniques

Pratyhara: focusing inward, withdrawing all your senses

Dharana: concentration

Dhyana: meditation

Samadhi: enlightenment

Clearly, Patanjali was incredibly wise because the concepts he laid out in his *Yoga Sutras* over 5,000 years ago are still quite relevant and important to our lives today. Think of them as a personal code of ethics—not commandments. It's important to understand that these eight limbs are *guidelines* to help you connect with your inner self and the more you put each facet into practice the closer you'll be to finding your life's purpose. Let's look at each of the limbs in more depth.

Limb 1: Yamas

The first limb is based on our ethics and is often guided by our moral compass. In other words: "Do unto others, as you would have others do unto you."

The 5 Yamas:

Ahimsa—non-violence. This is probably the most well-known yama, as it's the reason that most yogis become vegan or vegetarian. The practice of 'ahimsa' means that we do not harm (physically, emotionally, mentally) any other living thing. Yes, including animals. One of the keys to practicing ahimsa is learning to be more compassionate to others and ourselves.

Satya—truthfulness. The practice of satya means living and speaking the truth. However, it's much more difficult than it may seem—especially if you're following ahimsa. However, be mindful when speaking the truth so that you don't intentionally cause harm to another.

Asteya—non-stealing. When you look at the definition of asteya it might seem relatively simple to follow. However it's much more complex than just not stealing someone else's stuff. Asteya not only means that you shouldn't take what isn't given to you, but also that you shouldn't condone the behavior in others. In society this might mean being against oppression, injustices or exploitation in any way.

Brahmacharya—continence. This yama states that we should learn to separate ourselves from addictions and excess. Brahmacharya says that we should exercise control over our physical impulses and by doing so we become much healthier, wiser and stronger. By practicing moderation we learn to conserve our energy for what's most important—finding our true purpose in life.

Aparigraha—non-covetousness. When we look at the practice of Aparigraha it states that we should only keep what's necessary. This yama promotes minimalism and love for our true self. When we are constantly focused on attaining the newest and best material possession we lose sight of what's most important—enlightenment and purpose.

Practicing the five Yamas is in no way easy. It takes hard work and vigilance—especially in this day and age. However, it's not about being perfect and never making a mistake, but rather that you're striving to be the best version of yourself possible. By engaging in these practices you will strengthen your fortitude and character and inspire others to do the same.

Limb 2: Niyamas

Patanjali's second limb of yoga is referred to as the 'Niyamas.' Basically, this limb offers guidance on how you treat yourself. Hint: it's all about respect.

The 5 Niyamas:

Saucha—purification. In reference to the body it's fairly easy to see what Patanjali is talking about here. The practice of saucha refers to keeping our minds, bodies and environment as clean as possible. Why? In ancient yogic culture they discovered that when our internal environment (bodies) and external environment are cluttered, dirty, impure—then it's hard for us to reach enlightenment and inner peace. This goes for what we eat & drink, the company we keep, what we choose to entertain ourselves with, the music we listen to, etc. The goal is to not fill our bodies or minds with any form of impurities or uncleanliness.

Santosha—contentment. When we practice santosha, essentially we are teaching ourselves to be happy with what we've got. Think about the possibilities:

If we were happy with what we have, right now—the economy would collapse and we'd all be truly happy. I know it doesn't seem possible, but when we seek happiness through possessions we will always be disappointed. Every single time. If you practice being content then you have freed yourself from unneeded suffering and pain and will experience an influx of gratitude for the life that we do have.

Tapas—asceticism. No, I'm not talking about the Spanish cuisine. This kind of 'tapas' actually refers to the practice of self-discipline and doing things you don't want to do *right now* that will ultimately have a positive effect on your life in the future. Ancient yogis believed that by practicing this form of will power an internal "fire" is ignited within us. In turn it causes us to release dormant kundalini energy that ultimately helps us gain control over our unconscious impulses and behaviors.

Svadhyaya—self-study. The fourth niyama in Patanjali's *Sutra* is the ability to look deep within ourselves to assess our true nature through all the information we've gathered throughout our lives up until now.

The practice of svadhyaya allows us to examine and learn from our mistakes and weaknesses because we are always growing and changing. When we practice the art of self-study it allows us to see beyond the current moment and connect with the divine.

Ishvara Pranidhana—devotion. This niyama is the practice of giving up our egocentric identities and realizing that *we* are not *our body*—we just live in it. Ishvara can be seen as a sort of offering of the best things about ourselves to a higher power through which we grow in peace, grace and love.

Are you feeling overwhelmed yet? Yeah, I thought so. I realize this can be a lot of information to take in and it's kind of suffocating. But the good news is: again, these are *guidelines*. No one's expecting you to master all of these at once within a week. It takes a lifetime of practice to attain true spiritual enlightenment, but as long as you're trying that's half the battle.

To make things simple try practicing *one* of the niyamas each week and focus just on that one task. I'm sure the results that you get from doing this experiment will inspire you to keep growing and striving for something better.

Limb 3: Asanas

The third limb of Patanjali's *Yoga Sutras* is the practice of the postures and poses. It is also the most widely known aspect of yoga—at least in Western culture. When you think 'yoga' you think 'poses,' right? This is what the focus of most yoga studio classes are in the West.

As a yogi it's easy to focus on just this one limb of Patanjali's *Sutra*. Oftentimes, it's the only one beginners know. But there's so much more to it than just contorting oneself into bendy positions.

How many times have you been reminded that you aren't enough? It happens multiple times every single day with the media and society's standards dictating what is and isn't beautiful and who is or isn't good enough.

With yoga, the beautiful thing is that you're enough. Right now. You don't have to prove anything to anyone to achieve greatness and attain beauty.

It's within you at this very moment and the asanas give us a way to unlock this beauty and greatness.

By doing asanas on a regular basis it challenges us to focus our minds and emotions on one common goal: coming together and uniting as one entity. This becomes a metaphor for how we relate to the Universe and all other living this. Yoga gives us a vehicle for connecting with something greater than ourselves.

Limb 4: Pranayama

This limb of the *Yoga Sutras* focuses on breath control and breathing techniques. It might not seem like a very important facet of yoga, but it's actually (in my opinion) the single most important factor in your yoga practice.

Breath control leads to mind control and this is evident when we look at our actions when we get angry or frustrated or scared. What happens to your breathing? Most likely your breathing got very shallow and erratic and at times it can even feel restricted. If we breathed this way all the time we wouldn't be very healthy or feel very calm. We would be in a constant state of anxiety—all because of our breath.

Are you convinced of its importance now? Good. Even more importantly, when we learn to properly control our breath we are also able to control our prana (or life energy). By doing this we actually begin to restore and keep up with our health. In other words, we create balance in our bodies, which is vital to our happiness and overall well-being.

And just to illustrate how intelligent Patanjali was when he created the *Yoga Sutras* let's take a look at the pranayama and the asanas. They go hand in hand, right? It isn't considered a proper yoga asana if you aren't also incorporating the proper breathing techniques at the same time. But did you know that by performing the two together it creates 'tapas' within us—or internal heat—that helps to purify our bodies and minds? It's amazing how all of this fits together so well, isn't it? Patanjali was definitely a wise dude and knew what he was talking about.

Limb 5: Pratyahara

Pratyahara is sometimes one of the most confusing limbs of the ashtanga yoga practice. There are a lot of differing opinions as to what it actually refers to and how you can incorporate it into your yoga practice.

For me, the definition of pratyahara—which means focusing inward and suppressing your senses—isn't meant to be utilized in each moment of everyday life. I believe that Patanjali's original intentions for pratyahara was to disengage our senses when we're meditating or when we're practicing mindfulness.

In other words, if you're sweeping the floor—focus on *just sweeping the floor.* Or if you're talking to your significant other, focus on *just talking to your significant other.* It's easy for us to get distracted. Especially in this day and age, what with our smart phones, wi-fi everywhere, apps for everything, advertisements trying to steal our attention and a multitude of other attention stealers.

In relation to your yoga practice it's easier to think of it in terms of each pose. When you're doing a specific asana (for instance, savasana) the importance is to focus on only that pose and the movements or lack thereof it's comprised of. The challenge in savasana is shutting our minds off and focusing on relaxing every minute little muscle and tense part of our bodies. Think of it as a form of meditation if that makes it easier.

So the ultimate take-away from the practice of pratyahara is this: keep a buffer between your actions and the rest of the world. By putting pratyahara into effect it helps us avoid the knee-jerk reactions that we often use out of anger or assumption and instead gives us time to *choose* how to respond. Focusing on our ability to choose instead of letting our emotions dictate how we react—that's pratyahara.

Limb 6: Dharana

Although it's often overlooked, the practice of dharana is actually quite vital to a successful yoga journey. But what is it? Well, in layman's terms it simply means 'concentration.'

Basically the goal here is to focus your mind and attention on one single object or thought. If you're just starting out it's much easier to pick an object to practice on rather than a thought. However, "easy" is a misleading word for this particular exercise. As simple as the idea of dharana sounds it's actually quite difficult to be able to shut your mind off and focus on this one object.

The best way to start is by setting a timer for 10 minutes or so. Even 5 if you feel like 10 minutes is too much. Once your timer is set and you have your object of focus, get to work. Or rather, let your mind concentrate on the facets of the object you've chosen.

You might find that, in the beginning, your thoughts are going to wander. A lot. But don't worry: this is normal. Each time a random thought pops into your head, steering you away from the chosen object, gently guide your mind back to the original desired thought. At first this will happen constantly. However, over time you'll begin to notice that the more you practice the art of concentration, the better you'll become.

Once you've learned to purify your mind through the practice of concentration you will have mastered a skill that most people won't even come close to and you'll have the power to heal yourself in ways you never thought were possible.

Not to mention, if you're the kind of person who feels like their thoughts are constantly scattered and focused on multiple different ideas and tasks at once you'll start to appreciate the tranquility of being able to focus on one thing at a time.

Limb 7: Dhyana

Dhyana, or meditation, is the seventh limb of ashtanga yoga and is also quite commonly known in our culture. However, probably not in the sense that Patanjali envisioned it.

Dhyana and dharana tend to go hand in hand. You can't really have one without the other. So although these practices are learned separately, in daily use generally they're going to be combined together.

The practice of meditation is the ability to completely shut your mind off from any distractions or thoughts—to be utterly at peace. And it's definitely no simple task. If you thought dharana was difficult then be prepared for lots of practice with meditation. When we learn to fine-tune our mind's concentration we also become aware of the divine and our fears begin to vanish.

Later on in the book we'll talk more about how to actually utilize meditation and some easy(ish) strategies for developing a strong concentration and meditation habit.

Limb 8: Samadhi

The eighth and final limb is the sate of Samadhi, or enlightenment. I would say that this is the most intimidating practice outlined by Patanjali in his *Sutra's*—at least for me in the beginning.

And with good reason. I mean, after all, it's the *ultimate* goal of yoga—to experience enlightenment and super-consciousness. That's not intimidating at all, right?

When we actively achieve samadhi, all of our body's senses are at rest—as if we're asleep, yet our minds are awake and alert. This experience is truly divine and it awakens our unconscious mind in a way that was never achievable up until now.

We no longer feel tied to worldly concerns or material possessions—we have progressed beyond that to a realm of spiritual elation and liberation. When we're in the state of enlightenment we no longer distinguish between our self and non-self—it all becomes one elative experience.

Because samadhi is a difficult undertaking, it's best to start with proper preparation of your mind and body to get yourself in a peak state. There's a reason Patanjali laid the eight limbs out in the order that he did—it's a symbol of progression.

If you're going to attempt to reach enlightenment it's a good idea to start out with asanas and pranayama first and then move on to dharana, dhyana and finally samadhi.

By following Patanjali's progression through the eight-fold path it's much easier to attain a physical, emotional, ethical and spiritual state of being.

The Modern Yogic Body

So now that you've been primed on *what* exactly Patanjali's definition of yoga is—what does it all mean for **you**? I mean, it *was* written over 5,000 years ago. How relevant can it be to your life today?

I think if you've read over the Eight Limbs of Yoga it's pretty obvious when you apply it to your modern day yoga journey it still fits *scarily* well. The tradition of yoga kind of reminds me of a kite, lazily drifting on the breeze. It doesn't try to fight the wind or go in a different direction—yet somehow it always gets where it was meant to all along. That's what the tradition of yoga has done over all these years and throughout so many different cultures; it has presented itself exactly as it is, but it's been perceived and received in exactly the right ways and at exactly the right times.

This all might sound a little confusing, but really I'm just saying all this to get the point across that yoga is whatever you need it to be. And the modern yogi can be whatever she or *he* wants to be—on and off the mat.

The beauty of yoga is that there are no "rules." You have the freedom to be who you truly are and yoga helps you discover that person without asking for anything in return.

Okay, so we've covered the philosophy of yoga, but what about the physical body in regards to yoga? In this chapter we're going to go over our Koshas, Doshas and Chakras and what role they play in helping us unlock our purpose and potential on our yoga journey. Hint: it goes much deeper than looking good in a bikini.

5 Koshas, 5 Layers of Being

We'll start with our Koshas. The word 'kosha' actually translates to sheath. So when we talk about the koshas it's easiest to envision them each as a layer, or a sort of cloak of energy that we wear that transitions from our deep spiritual core to our outermost layer of skin—all of which to say it's basically a way for us to easily conceptualize ourselves. If we desire to live a completely balanced and healthy life (as most of us do) then we need to look at each of our bodies (or koshas) as their own entities and take care of them accordingly to ensure that things are running smoothly.

Annamaya kosha (Physical Body)—This is the body, or kosha, that we tend to spend the most time in. The translation translates literally to 'made of food.' This layer represents our physical body and is made up of our skin, tissues, fat, muscles and bones. This is where we engage with our physical senses—sight, smell, touch, taste and sound. The annamaya kosha is the only sheath that is made up of matter—the four others are states of energy and can't be detected with the human eye.

Pranamaya kosha (Energy Body)—The second layer of our koshas—the pranamaya refers to our prana, or life force. In traditional Chinese medicine this energy is referred to as chi. When we participate in certain homeopathy treatments like acupuncture we are actually targeting our energy body and aren't directly affecting our physical body.

In regards to yoga, this layer is what holds our physical body together—it regulates all of our biological processes like circulation, digestion and even breathing. The pranamaya kosha is what dictates our state of health and being. Without it we couldn't survive for more than a few minutes. There is a whole school of yoga devoted to replenishing our energy body—it's called pranayama and it focuses on diaphragmatic breathing exercises and alternate nostril breath techniques. To keep your prana in good working order you must get lots of sunshine and fresh air, which can also be found in fresh and organic whole foods.

Manomaya kosha (Emotional Body)—The third layer of our mental body is in charge of our reflexive and sensory functions. Basically, the manomaya kosha (which translates to 'body made of thought processes') handles the information we get from our five senses and responds for us without us even having to think about it—it's all automatic. When we're responding to our environment instead of making specific life choices we are aware of our emotional body.

In yogic culture, the brain and nervous system are viewed as the command center through the manomaya kosha and it dictates how our physical body responds to a given situation.

If you want to strengthen your manomaya kosha then practice mantra meditation on a regular basis, as this helps to soothe and balance this layer of our koshas by getting rid of negative energy pockets that prevent us from being at peace. Also, because our mental body is supplied by our senses, if we constantly bombard our third kosha with negative or violent forms of entertainment then we will create mental agitation within ourselves that leaves us unbalanced, which is why the regular practice of pratyahara (the 5th limb of yoga) is very important.

Vijnanamaya kosha (Wisdom Body)—Our fourth layer is made up of our wisdom body, or vijnanamaya kosha (which means 'the power of judgment or discernment'). This sheath is responsible for controlling our will and conscience. For instance, if you are lacking power in your wisdom body you may find that you lack strong values or morals or that you are easily swayed by temptation when it comes to benefitting yourself and taking advantage of others.

You may also feel like you have no control over your life or the decisions that you're making—you feel like someone else is making up your mind for you. As humans, this is the differentiating layer that separates us from being merely animals. We are the only species on Earth that has the ability to be in control of our own lives without relying solely on instinct.

When you practice the yamas and niyamas in Patanjali's *Yoga Sutras,* you are actively strengthening your wisdom body. Another way to strengthen the fourth kosha is through the practice of Jnana yoga.

Anandamaya kosha (Bliss Body)—The fifth and final layer of our koshas refers to our spiritual body. For most of us, we are never able to develop the anandamaya kosha, but it should always remain the ultimate goal.

In yoga, it is the final step to reaching awareness of our highest Self. When people talk about having near-death experiences and reference a bright white light and a huge outpouring of unconditional love and wisdom, the anandamaya kosha is what they are experiencing.

If you want to try and awaken your bliss body then you can practice acts of service (this helps to open our hearts to others), bhakti yoga (this helps to open our hearts to the divine) and samadhi (this helps to open our hearts to our own spiritual being).

Just as a heads up, in a lot of the ancient yogic texts the five koshas are lumped into three parts: the gross body, the astral body and the causal body. If you see these three mentioned it's safe to assume that they're simply talking about your five koshas.

The 3 Doshas

So now that we have a better understanding of our physical and energetic bodies, let's talk about our doshas—or our mind-body type. In Ayurveda (the traditional healing system of India), it is believed that there are five elements that flow throughout nature and are present in every cell of our bodies. These elements are space, air, fire, water and earth. When they are combined in different ways they make up the three doshas—or energies that make up our specific constitutions. The doshas are responsible for the individual characteristics that make up our mind, body and soul. Through the proper practice of yoga we ensure that they stay balanced.

Each of us has a varying degree of each dosha, however there will usually be a more predominant dosha present. To get the most benefit from yoga, it's important to remember that you should focus your practice on catering to your specific mind-body dosha. I'm sure you're curious as to what exactly they are and how you can use yoga to develop your predominate dosha, right? Well, let's take a look.

Vata Dosha (Space & Air)—The Vata dosha is responsible for movement and is made up of space and air elements. This dosha promotes flexibility and creativity. But be careful, because if you're mind-body type is predominantly vata dosha, then you will be prone to overexertion, anxiety and fatigue and should avoid the more fast-paced forms of yoga (like vinyasa or flow) as it tends to aggravate Vata. If you're going to practice these types of yoga then move slowly and carefully and feel free to extend the amount of time that you hold the poses.

Grounding and calming poses are ideal for someone who is Vata, as these tend to reduce stress and anxiety. These types of poses include: Mountain, Tree, Warriors I & II as these are grounding and help you to build strength. Also, all types of forward bends that target the pelvis are beneficial to Vata dosha. The same goes for poses that focus on your thighs and lower back.

If you're predominately Vata dosha it's especially important for you to take your time when in Savasana. Plan to spend at least 20 minutes resting and recharging here in this pose. You'll also benefit from a structured routine.

Pitta Dosha (Fire & Water)—The pitta dosha is responsible for our metabolism and digestion and is made up of fire and water elements. If your Pitta is in balance then it helps to promote understanding and intelligence. However, if you're predominantly Pitta dosha then you have a tendency to overheat. It's best for you to avoid any form of yoga that causes lots of sweating—like Bikram.

Keep in mind that inversions generate a rush of heat to your head and Pitta doshas should avoid doing them for extended periods of time. Focus your attention, instead, on relaxing poses that help release heat from your body. Examples of cooling poses would be anything that opens your chest or compresses your solar plexus (i.e., Bridge, Bow, Fish, Cobra, Camel, Pigeon).

If you're looking for good standing poses then Pitta's benefit from poses that open up their hips—try Warrior, Half Moon or Tree poses.

Anything that's going to promote a calming, relaxing state of mind toward your yoga practice will be beneficial. Remember to be kind to yourself and avoid comparing yourself to others.

Kapha Dosha (Water & Earth)—The kapha dosha is responsible for our stability and structure and is made up of water and earth elements. If you're predominantly Kapha dosha then you have a lot of stamina and strength, however try to keep your doshas balanced because you'll start suffering from excessive weight or lethargy when you're not in balance.

You benefit most from an energizing and fast-pace yoga practice. You'll want to focus on challenging yourself and create lots of heat within your body—otherwise you tend to feel sluggish or cold. To counteract this, do flow sequences early in the morning (around 6-10 am), which will help to energize you for the rest of the day. It's also a good idea for you to practice bellows breath to help cleanse and energize your body.

For predominant Kaphas, standing poses are beneficial. Especially if you maintain each pose for an extended period of time—up to 20 breaths. You also do well with backbends and anything that helps open the chest and increase the prana in your body.

As I said before, remember that everyone has a different degree of each of the three doshas and they will continue to change and fluctuate during your lifetime.

It's important to keep in mind that they can and will become imbalanced by the different factors of your yogic lifestyle—whether it be your diet, health or illness and even your environment.

By utilizing and prescribing yourself the correct yoga practice based on your predominant dosha type then you're much more likely to create a deep level of connection between your mind, body and spirit.

The 7 Chakras

The final element of our modern yogic body is comprised of our chakras. So what in the world are chakras? Well, in traditional Sanskrit, the word chakra translates to 'disk' or 'wheel.' When we look at chakras in terms of Ayurvedic yoga and meditation they represent wheels of energy in our body.

Basically, chakras are thought to be spinning, vortex-like energy centers at various points in our body. There are seven major ones that most people know about and these are the ones we'll talk about below. They start at the base of the spine and go in a line all the way up to the top of the head. Although most people are somewhat familiar with our seven main chakras, most aren't aware that we actually have many minor chakras all throughout our body.

Each of our chakras contains invisible forces of energy (or prana) that help to keep our life force healthy and vibrant. Each chakra corresponds to specific nerve centers in our body that is composed of major organs, nerves and emotional, psychological and spiritual states of being.

35

It's easier to visualize our chakras if you think of them as rechargeable batteries that we can revitalize through cosmic energy in our atmosphere.

When they're running smoothly, our chakras provide a flow of energy throughout our physical body. However, sometimes they can become blocked due to health issues, emotional problems or simply stress. As you can imagine, when any of our chakras become blocked this can cause lots of problems because our life force (or prana) is always in motion and would be hindered to flow properly.

Keeping our chakras open and aligned is essential to the health and well-being of our modern yogic body. It might seem complicated right now, but as long as you practice awareness of each element of your body, mind, spirit and soul then you can keep things balanced and flowing properly.

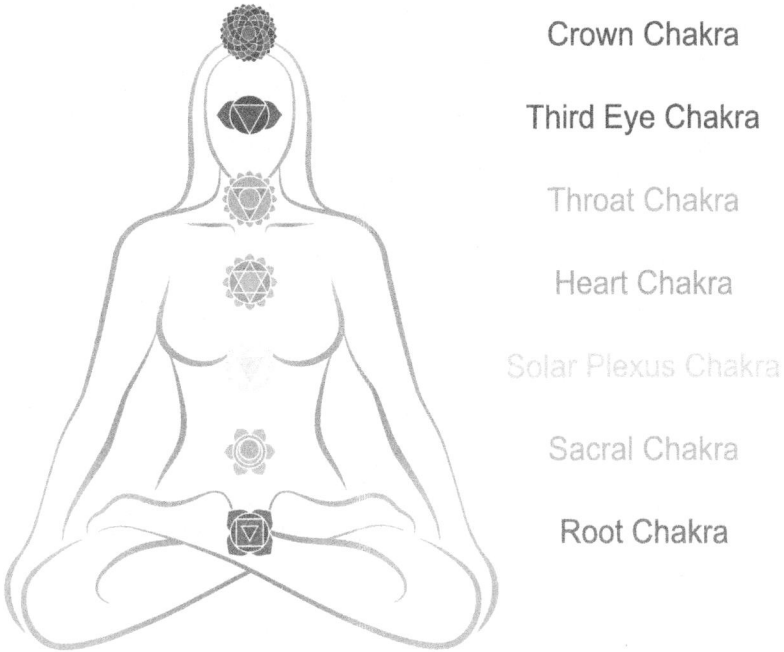

Crown Chakra

Third Eye Chakra

Throat Chakra

Heart Chakra

Solar Plexus Chakra

Sacral Chakra

Root Chakra

A diagram depicting the alignment of our 7 chakras.

The Root Chakra (Red)—Our root (or base) chakra is located at the base of our spine, encompassing our colon, bladder and first three vertebrae. This is also where our Kundalini energy is stored. This chakra is our most physical and because of this our energy tends to be rooted here.

When this chakra is out of balance you'll become greedy, almost voraciously so, fearful and overly emotional. However, when it's balanced you'll feel secure, calm and connected to the Earth.

Imbalances Cause: anemia, low back pain, sciatica, fatigue and depression. Also causes cold hands and feet.

Promotes Balance: restful sleep, physical exercise, working with your hands (i.e., building things, gardening, working with pottery), red foods & drinks, red clothing & gemstones, red oils (sandalwood, ylang ylang).

The Sacral Chakra (Orange)—The sacral (or spleen) chakra is our sexual and creativity center. It's located just above the pubic bone and below the navel. This chakra is connected to our emotions and how they relate to intimacy and social issues.

Imbalances Cause: anger, jealousy, codependency, eating disorders, depression, candida infections, UTIs, sexual impotence and drug and alcohol abuse.

Promotes Balance: massage, water aerobics, hot aromatherapy baths, focusing on pleasant sensations, orange foods & drinks, orange clothing & gemstones, orange oils (orange peel, melissa).

The Solar Plexus Chakra (Yellow)—The solar plexus chakra is the third chakra and is located just above our navel. It holds our source of personal power is where the center of our identity is kept and is how we relate to our higher selves.

The third chakra is in charge of our muscles, pancreas, adrenals and digestive system and is the seat of our emotional life.

When this chakra is in balance we have a very strong sense of self-esteem, responsibility, power and trust.

Imbalances Cause: emotional dysfunction (guilt, fear), constipation, toxicity, parasites, faulty memory, anxiety, ulcers, colitis, digestive problems, hypoglycemia and diabetes.

Promotes Balance: learning (reading, taking classes), doing brain teasers, sunshine, detox programs, yellow foods & drinks, yellow clothing & gemstones, yellow oils (rosemary, lemon).

The Heart Chakra (Green)—The heart chakra is located in, yep, you guessed it: the center of the chest over the heart. As is evident by its name, this chakra is responsible for our feelings of compassion, love, peace and harmony.

Because it's the exact center and connection point for all of our chakras it bridges our mind, body, spirit and emotions—it's our source of connection and love.

When the fourth chakra is in balance you become at peace with your environment, others and yourself.

Imbalances Cause: loneliness, resentment, heart & breast cancer, heart & breathing disorders, high blood pressure, chest pain, immune system issues, muscular tension and passivity.

Promotes Balance: socialization with family & friends, walks in nature, green foods & green drinks, green clothing & gemstones, green oils (pine, eucalyptus).

The Throat Chakra (Blue)—The throat chakra is quite fittingly located within your throat and it is considered the chakra of creativity, self-expression, communication and judgment. This fifth chakra includes your neck, jaw, mouth, tongue, thyroid and parathyroid glands of your body.

When the throat chakra is balanced there is purity of expression, speech and choice.

Imbalances Cause: addiction, criticism, bitterness, swollen glands, thyroid imbalances, infections, flu & fever, mouth/tongue/jaw/neck problems, hormone disorders, mood swings, hyperactivity, menopause and bloating.

Promotes Balance: poetry/writing, art collecting, singing in the shower, deep conversations, blue foods & drinks, blue clothing & gemstones, blue oils (geranium, chamomile).

The Brow Chakra (Indigo)—The brow chakra is often referred to as our third eye chakra. It is located right between our eyebrows and it's the center of our intuition. Many times we tend to ignore our intuition and focusing on opening your third eye will help you hone your ability to follow and "hear" your intuition more easily.

When there is balance in our sixth chakra the relationship that we have with our highest and spirit self are heightened.

Imbalances Cause: untruthfulness, depression, coordination problems, learning disabilities and sleep disorders.

Promotes Balance: meditation, stargazing, indigo foods & drinks, indigo clothing & gemstones, indigo oils (frankincense, patchouli).

The Crown Chakra (Violet)—The crown chakra is found at the very top of your head and is associated with our central nervous system, pituitary gland and also our cerebral cortex. It is seen as the charka of spiritual connection and enlightenment—through this chakra we are able to connect with our higher selves and also to the divine.

When the crown chakra is in balance you'll feel alive (physically and spiritually) and connected to the Universe. This is one of the most important chakras when you're trying to fulfill your life's purpose or destiny.

Imbalances Cause: selfishness, genetic disorders, psychological problems, headaches, neuralgia, coordination problems, epilepsy, senility, skin rashes, varicose veins and photosensitivity.

Promotes Balance: writing down goals and intentions, dream building, violet foods & drinks, violet clothing & gemstones, violet oils (jasmine, lavender).

Connecting All the Pieces

By utilizing all three parts of our yogic body—the Koshas, Doshas and Chakras— we can attain true spiritual awareness and become the healthiest version of ourselves possible.

Please keep in mind that, just like the 8 Limbs of Yoga, these are merely guidelines and sources of inspiration on your journey to betterment. You're never going to master every single practice or tap into each and every kosha and chakra all at once. No one expects you to be able to do that, either.

The point is merely that you are trying to attain enlightenment and are focused on becoming a better person than you were yesterday. If you're making progress then that's all you need to worry about.

The yogic lifestyle is incredibly flexible and open-minded to your interpretations of each practice and you absolutely *should* make them your own. If your personal third eye is guiding you to avoid a certain practice, listen to it! That's part of the process: figuring out what works for you and what doesn't.

Just like when you're talking about your predominant dosha—it's not going to be a one-size fits all experience. In fact, you might have two equally dominant doshas and that's perfectly okay. It happens. Go with the flow and don't stress.

The modern yogic body is comprised of many different elements that all work in harmony to enrich our lives in one way or another. As long as you're honoring your temple (your body) you'll get where you were meant to be.

The Modern Yogic Mind

Now that we've covered the need of our modern yogic body, it's time to focus on our modern yogic *mind*. The idea might sound somewhat intimidating, but I promise it's not all that bad and is quite accessible—even if you're a beginner.

When I refer to the yogic mind, I simply mean the practice of meditation and mindfulness as it relates to yoga. When the yogic mind, body and spirit are all interconnected properly you will be able to live without fear or anxiety of the unknown and will be free from pain and suffering.

So for this chapter we'll be looking at meditation and mindfulness and the how we can incorporate these practices into our yoga routine to help develop our higher selves.

If you think that meditation is in-accessible and unnecessary in this day and age and that you're simply just too busy to partake then I hate to break it to you, but you probably need it the most. Isn't that always how it works?

Hopefully by the end of this chapter you'll see that it's actually quite easy to do and you'll be able to find the perfect style of meditation that's right for you.

What is Meditation?

Well, for starters, Patanjali thought it was such an integral part of a healthy lifestyle and yoga journey that he assigned it as one of the eight limbs of yoga (Dhyana).

Generally speaking, I think that most of us make meditation way too complicated. After all, it's simply the act of sitting in silence and clearing your mind. Now, I hear you, at first it can be quite difficult to do and I'm probably making it out to be much easier than it actually is as a beginner. But I promise once you've practiced it enough, the habit will transform your mind and help to cultivate positivity and peace within you.

Benefits of Meditation

I'm sure you've heard many of the numerous reasons to practice meditation so I'll be brief, but I do think it's something that's worth repeating. Here are some things you can expect from making meditation a habit in your life.

- Increases your social connection and decreases feelings of loneliness
- Helps to develop laser sharp focus and attention
- Greater memory capabilities
- Gives you a higher level of self-esteem
- Decreases pain and inflammation in the body
- Improves your compassion and empathy toward others
- Reduces anxiety and depression
- Boosts gray matter and brain volume
- Increases feelings of gratitude

So basically...there's no reason *not* to start making meditation a daily part of your life. Right now. If you need help choosing which type of meditation will work best for you, then keep reading.

Finding Your "Om" Meditation Style

When most people think of meditation they simply think of mindfulness meditation, since that's what most beginners start out practicing. But did you know that there are many different styles of meditation and each one is as unique as you are?

In this chapter we're going to look at the eight main types of meditation and from there you can decide which one would work best for you. The good news is you don't have to stick to just one—you can pick and choose what works or doesn't depending on the day of the week.

Have fun with it and don't be too stressed about making a choice. After all, that kinda defeats the purpose, right? If it's helpful, try listening to your third eye chakra and let it guide you to a decision.

Popular Forms of Meditation

Mindfulness Meditation—As I stated before, this is probably one of the most common types of meditation practiced by beginners. It was first introduced in 1979 by Jon Kabat-Zinn and has since grown in popularity because it's so accessible in our everyday lives.

There are two techniques used here: breath awareness and body scan. For the first, you simply keep your attention on the inhalation and exhalation of your breath. For body scan, you focus your attention on your physical body—starting at your toes as you work your way up to your head.

This creates a higher state of awareness and ensures of the release of tension in all areas of your body.

Try it if... you are new to meditation.

Guided Meditation—This type of meditation is, as the name suggest, led by someone else. Generally it's a teacher or instructor and you would be part of a class. Usually there's a greater purpose to each class (i.e., relationship improvement, cultivating prosperity, awakening the chakras) but not always.

Many of the techniques used in guided meditation tend to vary between classes and teachers because most guided meditations will somewhat reflect the life experiences your "guide" has been influenced by.

I personally enjoy guided meditation, because it feels much easier for me to get in a state of serenity and peace when I don't have to do the thinking—someone else is calling the shots for me.

Try it if... you just want to sit back and relax.

Focused Meditation—This is a somewhat generalized form of meditation that simply refers to the act of focusing on one object or idea while turning your mind off to any other patterns of thinking that distract you from your focus.

Some people actually find this form of meditation easier than the practice of mindfulness since you're allowed to focus on anything you want that involves your senses.

Try it if... you want to break the multi-tasking habit.

Mantra Meditation—This type of meditation refers to the repetitive use of a single sound or set of sounds. By doing this you're able to go into and stay in a meditative state. This form of meditation has become popularized in movies and on television by the characteristic repetition of the 'om' sound.

Mantra meditation can help sharpen your focus and can be performed in various ways. Most of the time the sounds are chanted or whispered quietly. However, it's perfectly fine to say the phrase loudly if that's what feels best to you.

Try it if... you have a hard time sitting in silence.

Transcendental Meditation—The practice of transcendental meditation was popularized by certain celebrities, including the Beatles, Jennifer Aniston and supermodel Gisele Bundchen—just to name a few. As of today transcendental meditation is one of the most widely practiced forms of meditation (boasting over 6 million practitioners) and also one of the most frequently studied forms of meditation in research labs.

What is it? Well, it's simply the act of sitting comfortable with your eyes closed twenty minutes, twice a day. By doing so you learn to quiet your mind and experience a pure consciousness that was unattainable before.

Try it if... you like to go with the flow.

Kundalini Meditation—When most people hear 'kundalini' they think yoga. And yes, it's true that kundalini is a type of yoga. However, it's also an ancient yogic philosophy and name for a specific type of energy. Remember our chakras? Kundalini is said to lie coiled at our base (or root) chakra and becomes awakened as we tap into it—slowly rising up through each chakra, activating new waves of energy as it does.

When you practice kundalini meditation you use focus, mantras, mudras and your breath all in combination to push the coiled energy upward and by doing so you're able to change your state of mind to that of ecstasy.

This type of meditation, since it's so specific is best practiced with a teacher.

53

Try it if... you are interested in activating your chakras.

Zen (or Zazen)—The translation of Zazen means 'seated meditation,' which is fitting for the practice. Zen tends to focus on the philosophies that stem from Buddhist teachings.

The emphasis here is on attaining enlightenment through your breath techniques and mind and also from interaction with a teacher.

Try it if... you like guidelines and rules.

Primordial Sound Meditation—PSM is a type of silent meditation that focuses on the use of a mantra. It's believed to be a healing form of meditation that helps us to achieve deep relaxation and inner calm.

The mantra that is used in PSM is the specific vibration of the universe at the time and place you were born. It's actually calculated just for you using traditional Vedic math formulas.

By repeating this personal mantra that is yours only, it helps you to grow deeper within yourself to focus on comfort and better self-awareness.

This form of meditation was actually developed by Dr. Deepak Chopra and is the forms of meditation that they teach the Chopra Center.

Try it if... you like for things to be more personalized.

Sun Salutations

But what if you don't want to practice meditation and you simply just can't bring yourself to do it?

Well, I still think you should try it, but if you need to ease yourself into it then I recommend starting each morning with sun salutations, preferably outdoors facing the rising sun. If you're not familiar with what a sun salutation is, it's simply a series of yoga poses that are performed in a flow-type sequence. I'll show you how to perform a sun salutation on the next page.

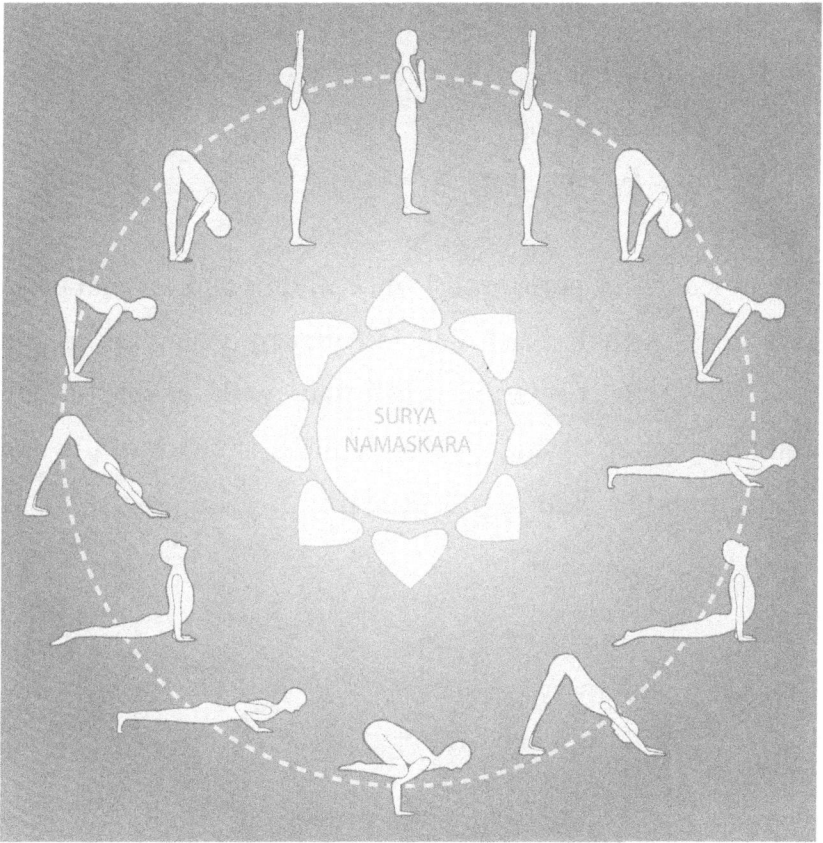

Here's an example of a more challenging sun salutation variation.

Generally speaking, each sun salutation (although they can vary) will have eight basic postures included:

- Mountain Pose
- Upward Salute
- Standing Forward Bend
- Lunge

57

- Plank Pose
- Four-Limbed Staff
- Upward-Facing Dog
- Downward-Facing Dog

The significance of performing sun salutations at a moderate or slow pace is that it helps to put you in a meditative and relaxed state. By beginning each day with a set of sun salutations you are easing your body into the chaos of life and giving your mind a chance to set the pace for your day.

Putting It Together

That wasn't so bad, now was it? You should now understand the inner workings of the modern yogic mind and what it takes to cultivate a life of harmony between your conscious and subconscious mind.

I also hope that you've found a form of meditation that sounds interesting to you and, more importantly, that you put it into practice.

If you still feel a little stuck on how to get started with your meditation habit, take baby steps. You don't have to (and shouldn't) start out with the goal of practicing Primordial Sound Meditation for 30 minutes every single day.

Start with just 2 minutes a day of a simple form of mindful meditation and you can work your way up after a week or two. The goal here is to simply take action—otherwise we tend to get wrapped up in the do's and don'ts and never get started.

The same is true for your sun salutations—just *do* them. It could be a round of three or even just one. The key is that you can go at your own pace without feeling any pressure or guilt about doing so.

Remember: the key to any aspect of a well-rounded yoga lifestyle is regularity and commitment. Without consistent discipline and practice you won't get very far.

Detoxifying Your Yogic Body

Remember how in the *Yoga Sutras* one of the five Niyamas was actually 'saucha'—or purification? Well, in this chapter that's exactly what we're going to talk about.

In order to keep our bodies and minds running at a peak state, it's extremely important that we also do our part to keep every aspect of our body as clean as possible. Literally and figuratively speaking.

There are quite a few ways that we can do this. For starters, we will look at the Shat Karmas, or six purifications.

The 6 Purifications

These six practices are thought to be one of the oldest rituals for self-cleansing and detoxification that exists. In ancient yogic culture, both physical and mental health were of utmost importance and by following these six steps of purification you would be able to heal virtually anything.

1. **Neti:** This is the process of cleaning out your nasal passages by using a small pot called a Neti pot. You can still find these in health food stores today and many people practice cleansing their nasal cavities with salt water to relieve sinusitis, headaches and allergies.

   The other form of this practice is called Sutra Neti in which a threaded is inserted into one nostril, pulled out the throat and out of the mouth. You then use a gentle flossing sort of motion to clean your nasal passage. Repeat for the other side.

2. **Dhauti:** This is the practice of cleaning one's stomach and is performed on an empty stomach, first thing in the morning. The process involves drinking 1 liter of saline water and then vomiting everything out. The purpose is remove undigested food that is still sitting in the stomach that will eventually cause digestion problems.

3. **Bhasti:** This practice refers to cleaning the bowels. In modern times we do this by inserting an enema tube into our anus to manually stimulate the cleansing of our colon. You can also get a colonic performed by a professional if you don't feel comfortable administering an enema.

4. **Nauli:** Practicing Nauli means churning your abdominal muscles repeatedly to the right and then left. By doing this you rotate your muscles and tone up all your organs preventing digestive disorders. This is one of the more difficult purifications to master.

5. **Kapalabhati:** This process is often referred to as a type of pranayama. It's a breathing technique that cleans the lungs by forcefully expelling the air and getting rid of any accumulated carbon dioxide left in our lungs. You repeat this process several times, forcefully expelling the air, while breathing in normally.

6. **Trataka:** When one practices Trataka it helps to develop concentration and get rid of anxiety. The mechanics of it are fairly simple: you focus on a single point without blinking your eyes, which is thought to improve eyesight and promote clarity of the mind.

Although these practices are somewhat outdated now, there is still some truth to following a ritual like this on a weekly, monthly or seasonal basis. The good news is, though, that there are many more easily accessible ways of cleansing our bodies without having to induce vomiting or thread a string through your nasal passages.

Modern Day Detox

So what does a modern day detox ritual look like? Well, it's really going to depend on the person and his or her specific needs. However, there are some basic habits that most of us can all benefit from at some point or another.

Here are some ideas to get you started...

Juicing—Incorporating juicing should be a daily practice in your life already. If you haven't gotten on the juice train yet, you should start now. However, when I say juice I don't mean pure fruit juice. I'm referring to mostly green veggie juice. It's actually pretty tasty and it's the fastest way to get a super-concentrated amount of nutrients into your blood stream.

Fasting—This form of detox has many different variations and is really up to your own personal discretion. You can choose to either do a juice fast or a water fast, but if you're just starting out I recommend sustaining yourself with juice as you'll be able to function much easier. Fasting can be done twice a year for two weeks at a time. Or, you can do it with each change of the seasons for a week at a time. You could even simply dedicate one day a week to refrain from eating. This is known as intermittent fasting and it has major health benefits—the main one being an increase in the longevity of your life.

Raw Food Diet—This is a somewhat easy way to detox from all the fast food and processed stuff that we eat on a regular basis. If you're finding it hard to break free from food addiction, then a raw food diet would be a great way to heal your body and detox from the inside out. A good starting point would be trying one raw meal a day or if you're feeling adventurous, commit to one month of raw eating.

Dry Brushing—This is one of the easiest ways to cleanse your body and stimulate your lymph system. At any health food store purchase a dry brush and simply use it once a day, or at least weekly, to remove dead skin cells and stimulate re-growth before showering.

Colon Cleansing—Generally we refer to this detox practice as an enema, but you can also schedule an appointment with a professional to get a colonic in which they irrigate your colon for you in a less intimidating manner. There are many amazing health benefits to cleansing your colon regularly, but the main one is that it aids in the removal of toxins and waste products that have built up in your body and can't find a way out. Just remember if you perform an enema or get a colonic to take probiotics to help restore the healthy gut flora.

Epsom Salt Baths—This one is really easy as well! Simply fill up your bathtub with as-hot-as-you-can-stand-it water and dump in a few cups of epsom salts before getting in. Soak in the water for around 20 minutes or so.

Not only is it just nice for your body and mind to get to relax for a while, but it also promotes the relief of inflammation and muscle cramps as well as the removal of heavy metals and toxins from our cells—along with lots of other benefits. Just be careful not to stay in too long because the combination of the rush of magnesium into your body and hot water can cause dizziness and fatigue.

Parasite Cleansing—Surprisingly, not many of us do this and unfortunately it's one of the most important methods of detoxification and cleansing we can experience. This paragraph isn't big enough for me to go on about the dangers and negative health affects caused by parasites (I really need to write a book about it!), but I can assure you every single one of us has them and could live with far less. They rob us of our vital life nutrients and even take our brains hostage. If you haven't performed a parasite cleanse in the last 6 months you need to do one now!

Restorative Yoga—Here's an easy one. Restorative yoga is incredibly beneficial for assisting in the process of detoxification of our minds and bodies. If you're not familiar with this type of yoga, I'll break it down for you: it's basically the most relaxing style of yoga there is and it promotes quieting of the mind and overall stress reduction. If you're feeling burnt out with your yoga practice or current exercise routine, I recommend giving restorative yoga a try—it's basically adult naptime.

Massage Therapy—I'm sure we all know how great getting a massage *feels* but did you know it actually has major health benefits? It's true. So the next time your husband says you can't afford to get a massage, rattle off how healing and detoxifying it can be for your entire body and mind. Once you know how healthy it is for you, it goes from a luxury to a necessity.

Acupuncture—This practice originated in China and involves the Acupuncturist inserting extremely thin needles into specific points in a patient's skin. I know it doesn't sound very pleasant, but it's actually quite invigorating and if you haven't tried it you should give it a go. Remember when we talked about the five koshas? Acupuncture actually helps you to target and focus in on your pranayama kosha and can even get rid of chronic pain. If you've been curious about it, but just haven't given it a chance I urge you to take the leap and experience the relief that it can provide.

You definitely won't regret it.

So from the six purifications all the way up to modern forms of detoxification, you should now be an expert on cleansing your body and mind. Again, as with all the information in this book these are just meant to provide inspiration and be a sort of guideline to push you forward along your journey.

Maybe you aren't quite ready to make colon cleansing part of your routine—I get it. It can be scary and a little weird. Just take it at your own pace.

Like anything, start out small and work your way up. Don't get overwhelmed by the numbers of choices and remain stagnant. Any form of change is good, no matter how minute it might seem to you.

Now that you've got your yogic body and mind under control and are in the detox phase, let's see how it all fits together and helps you to fulfill your life's purpose.

Living Your Purpose

The bigger picture of yoga is a lifestyle. There is no one path that's right or no one path that's wrong. That's one of my favorite things about yoga: it gives you the freedom and ability to be who you *truly* are. There's not much in life that you can say that about.

Most things in our society try to shape us or make us up into who *they* think we should be. Fit us into *their* definition of pretty. And then if they can't do that or we refuse, there's something wrong with *us*. Well, I'm here to tell you that yoga can be your safe place. It can be all the things that you ever wanted or dreamed it could be.

There's just one catch: you have to be vulnerable and believe in the power of change. Your yoga journey isn't going to be a smooth ride. There's going to be bumps and roadblocks and crazy emotional outbursts—but guess what?

That's all normal. We've all been there. And if you are brave enough to keep pushing and come out on the other side, you'll be rewarded with a sense of awareness and gratitude that most never get to experience.

Why is all this important? Well, when we feel there's no direction in our lives or it lacks meaning then we start to feel depressed and isolated from the rest of the world and our Creator. If there's no connection or vibrancy or if we don't feel enthusiastic about anything then we tend to ask ourselves 'What's the point?' And for good reason: our higher Self *knows* that there's more out there. Just like you *knew* there was more to yoga than just some challenging poses—and the same reasons you picked up this book.

Call it your third eye or your intuition—whatever you want to call it, there's a reason you're feeling the way that you are. If you find it extremely hard to get out of bed every morning and are depressed at the idea of going to a job you hate—there's a reason for that as well. Maybe you simply don't find your work rewarding or enriching to your life.

If that's the case, don't keep making excuses for yourself—find something you *love* doing more than anything else. Maybe you know what that passion is at this very moment. Do you like to design t-shirts? Are you into drawing comics?

Do you find it rewarding to serve others? Whatever it is that you love to do, more than anything—I'm talking love-it-so-much-I'd-do-it-for-free kind of love—then pursue *that*. Find a way to make *that* a career.

No matter how silly your dream or passion may be to someone else or how crazy it seems to ditch a job making five times more money—deep down you know it's the right thing to do.

In the end, the amount of material possessions or monetary gains we've accomplished aren't going to matter. We can't take that stuff with us. What's truly important? The level of happiness we experience on a daily basis, how we make others feel, whether or not we are inspiring change in the world and upholding our own personal morals.

I'm sure you know most of this already—like I said, it's intuitive. But the thing is: if we know this stuff, why don't we take action on it?

Instead, we continue to do the things day in and day out that make us so incredibly unhappy. And for what—money? Status? Fear of change or the unknown? Maybe we feel like we don't truly deserve to be happy.

If that's the case, then it just goes to show why it's so important that our mind-body connection is in tune and working together. When things are off balance we tend to feel less-than and uninspired to do good things. Often times we feel incapable and doubt ourselves.

This is just a friendly reminder that, even though it's not easy, it's definitely worth fighting and striving for a sense of purpose in the world. When you discover what it is and are brave enough to accept the journey that lies ahead of you, there is no doubt that you'll harvest a lifetime of happiness and karma that will be repaid to you ten-fold for generations to come, and who knows, maybe you'll even reach anandamaya kosha.

Conclusion

This journey that we call life is a crazy one—especially in this modern age of technology. There are so many things that attempt to compromise our well-being and personal code of ethics.

I think this is why a yogic lifestyle is so important—no matter who you are there's great benefit to striving for more. Like I've said over and over again: this lifestyle is going to look different for everyone. There are going to be discrepancies, but it's more about how it all makes you *feel.* Just like when you're in an asana—your focus should be on the feeling you get, not how you look.

The practice of yoga has given me, and so many others amazing insight into the roots of humanity and helped countless men and women discover a much greater divine purpose. Now, I'm not saying I'm religious and I'm not saying you need to be in order to live out a yogic lifestyle, but be prepared because it does change you for the better from the inside out into someone you never knew you could be.

It gives you the empowerment that you may have lacked before to really free your body, mind and spirit of the societal constraints that we often face in these modern times.

I know that I don't have all the answers—I'm just a mere human like you are—but I do know that wherever you want to go in life, or whoever you want to be...yoga can take you there or shape you into that. You just have to give it the chance.

Love and light,
Olivia

Printed in Great Britain
by Amazon

39222912R00046